Ketogenic Air Fryer

Unmissable Recipes

Boost Your Metabolism and Enjoy Your

Meals with Incredibly Tasty Ketogenic Air

Fryer Dishes

Nolan Turner

advice. The content within this book has been derived from various sources. Please consult a licensed professional before attempting any techniques outlined in this book.

By reading this document, the reader agrees that under no circumstances is the author responsible for any losses, direct or indirect, which are incurred as a result of the use of information contained within this document, including, but not limited to, — errors, omissions, or inaccuracies.

Table of Contents

Walnut Bars

Preparation time: 5 minutes **Cooking time**: 16 minutes **Servings**: 4

Ingredients:

1 egg

1/3 cup cocoa powder 3 tablespoons swerve

7 tablespoons ghee, melted 1 teaspoon vanilla extract

¼ cup almond flour

¼ cup walnuts, chopped

½ teaspoon baking soda

Directions:

In a bowl, mix all the ingredients and stir well. Spread this on a baking sheet that fits your air fryer lined with parchment paper, put it in the fryer and cook at 330 degrees F and bake for 16 minutes. Leave the bars to cool down, cut and serve.

Nutrition: calories 182, fat 12, fiber 1, carbs 3, protein 6

Aromatic Cup

Prep time: 10 minutes **Cooking time:** 15 minutes
Servings: 1

Ingredients:

1 egg, beaten

1 tablespoon peanut butter

½ teaspoon baking powder

1 teaspoon lemon juice

½ teaspoon vanilla extract

1 teaspoon Erythritol

2 tablespoons coconut flour

Directions:

Mix up all ingredients in the cup until homogenous. Then preheat the air fryer to 350F. Put the cup with blondies in the air fryer and cook it for 15 minutes.

Nutrition: calories 237, fat 15, fiber 7, carbs 14, protein 12.6

Chocolate Ramekins

Preparation time: 5 minutes **Cooking time**: 15 minutes **Servings**: 6

Ingredients:

cup blackberries

eggs

½ cup heavy cream

½ cup ghee, melted

¼ cup chocolate, melted 1 tablespoons stevia

2 teaspoons baking powder

Directions:

In a bowl, mix the blackberries with the rest of the ingredients, whisk well, divide into ramekins, put them in the fryer and cook at 340 degrees F for 15 minutes. Serve cold.

Nutrition: calories 150, fat 2, fiber 2, carbs 4, protein 7

Cocoa Spread

Prep time: 10 minutes **Cooking time:** 5 minutes
Servings: 4

Ingredients:

2 oz walnuts, chopped

5 teaspoons coconut oil

½ teaspoon vanilla extract

1 tablespoon Erythritol

1 teaspoon of cocoa powder

Directions:

Preheat the air fryer to 350F. Put the walnuts in the mason jar. Add coconut oil, vanilla extract, Erythritol, and cocoa powder. Stir the mixture until smooth with the help of the spoon. Then place the mason jar with Nutella in the preheated air fryer and cook it for 5 minutes. Stir Nutella before serving.

Ginger Vanilla Cookies

Preparation time: 10 minutes **Cooking time**: 15 minutes **Servings**: 12

Ingredients:

2 cups almond flour 1 cup swerve

¼ cup butter, melted 1 egg

2 teaspoons ginger, grated 1 teaspoon vanilla extract

¼ teaspoon nutmeg, ground

¼ teaspoon cinnamon powder

Directions:

In a bowl, mix all the ingredients and whisk well. Spoon small balls out of this mix on a lined baking sheet that fits the air fryer lined with parchment paper and flatten them. Put the sheet in the fryer and cook at 360 degrees F for 15 minutes. Cool the cookies down and serve.

Nutrition: calories 220, fat 13, fiber 2, carbs 4, protein 3

Vanilla Mozzarella Balls

Prep time: 20 minutes **Cooking time:** 4 minutes **Servings:** 8

Ingredients:

2 eggs, beaten

1 teaspoon almond butter, melted

7 oz coconut flour

2 oz almond flour

5 oz Mozzarella, shredded

1 tablespoon butter

2 tablespoons swerve

1 teaspoon baking powder

½ teaspoon vanilla extract

Cooking spray

Directions:

In the mixing bowl mix up butter and Mozzarella. Microwave the mixture for 10-15 minutes or until it is melted. Then add almond flour and coconut flour. Add swerve and baking powder. After this, add vanilla extract and stir the mixture. Knead the soft dough. Microwave the mixture for 2-5 seconds more if it is not melted enough. In the bowl mix up almond butter and eggs. Make 8 balls from the almond flour mixture and coat them in the egg mixture. Preheat the air fryer to 400F. Spray the air fryer basket with cooking spray from inside and place the bread rolls in one layer.

Cook the dessert for 4 minutes or until the bread roll is golden brown. Cool the cooked dessert completely and sprinkle with Splenda if desired.

Nutrition: calories 249, fat 14.4, fiber 10.9, carbs 8.3, protein 13.3

Avocado Salad

Prep time: 10 minutes **Cooking time:** 3 minutes
Servings: 4

Ingredients:

1 avocado, peeled, pitted and roughly sliced

½ teaspoon minced garlic

¼ teaspoon chili flakes

½ teaspoon olive oil

1 tablespoon lime juice

¼ teaspoon salt

1 teaspoon cilantro, chopped

1 cup baby spinach

1 cup cherry tomatoes halved

Cooking spray

Directions:

Preheat the air fryer to 400F. Then spray the air fryer basket with cooking spray from inside. Combine all the ingredients inside, cook for 3 minutes, divide into bowls and serve.

Nutrition: calories 142, fat 10.2, fiber 2.7, carbs 4.9, protein 8.8

Cheddar Kale Mix

Preparation time: 5 minutes **Cooking time**: 20 minutes **Servings**: 4

Ingredients:

½ cup black olives, pitted and sliced 1 cup kale, chopped

tablespoons cheddar, grated 4 eggs, whisked

Cooking spray

A pinch of salt and black pepper

Directions:

In a bowl, mix the eggs with the rest of the ingredients except the cooking spray and whisk well. Grease a pan that fits the air fryer with the cooking spray, pour the olives mixture inside, spread, put the pan into the machine, and cook at 360 degrees F for 20 minutes. Serve for breakfast hot.

Nutrition: calories 220, fat 13, fiber 4, carbs 6, protein 12

Mozzarella Swirls

Prep time: 15 minutes **Cooking time:** 12 minutes
Servings: 6

Ingredients:

2 tablespoons almond flour

1 tablespoon coconut flour

½ cup Mozzarella cheese, shredded

1 teaspoon Truvia

2 tablespoons butter, softened

¼ teaspoon baking powder

1 egg, beaten

Cooking spray

Directions:

In the bowl mix up almond flour, coconut flour, Mozzarella cheese, Truvia, butter, baking powder, and egg. Knead the soft and non-sticky dough. Then preheat the air fryer to 355F. Meanwhile, roll up the cheese dough and cut it into 6 pieces. Make the swirl from every dough piece.

Spray the air fryer basket with cooking spray. Place the cheese swirls in the air fryer in one layer and cook them for 12 minutes or until they are light brown. Repeat the same step with remaining uncooked dough. It is recommended to serve the cheese Danish warm.

Nutrition: calories 115, fat 10, fiber 2, carbs 3.9, protein 4

Tomatoes Casserole

Preparation time: 5 minutes **Cooking time**: 15 minutes **Servings**: 4

Ingredients:

4 eggs, whisked

1 teaspoon olive oil

3 ounces Swiss chard, chopped 1 cup tomatoes, cubed

Salt and black pepper to the taste

Directions:

In a bowl, mix the eggs with the rest of the ingredients except the oil and whisk well. Grease a pan that fits the fryer with the oil, pour the swish chard mix and cook at 359 degrees F for 15 minutes. Divide between plates and serve for breakfast.

Nutrition: calories 202, fat 14, fiber 3, carbs 5, protein 12

Creamy Chives Muffins

Prep time: 15 minutes **Cooking time:** 12 minutes
Servings: 4

Ingredients:

4 slices of ham

¼ teaspoon baking powder

4 tablespoons coconut flour

4 teaspoons heavy cream

1 egg, beaten

1 teaspoon chives, chopped

1 teaspoon olive oil

½ teaspoon white pepper

Directions:

Preheat the air fryer to 365F. Meanwhile, mix up baking powder, coconut flour, heavy cream, egg, chives, and white pepper. Stir the ingredients until getting a smooth mixture. Finely chop the ham and add it in the muffin liquid. Brush the air fryer muffin molds with olive oil. Then pour the muffin batter in the molds. Place the rack in the air fryer basket and place the molds on it. Cook the muffins for 12 minutes (365F). Cool the muffins to the room temperature and remove them from the molds.

Nutrition: calories 125, fat 7.8, fiber 3.5, carbs 6.1, protein 7.7

Salmon and Spinach Scramble

Preparation time: 5 minutes **Cooking time**: 20 minutes **Servings**: 4

Ingredients:

A drizzle of olive oil

1 spring onion, chopped

1 cup smoked salmon, skinless, boneless and flaked 4 eggs, whisked

A pinch of salt and black pepper

¼ cup baby spinach

4 tablespoon parmesan, grated

Directions:

In a bowl, mix the eggs with the rest of the ingredients except the oil and whisk well. Grease the Air Fryer with the oil, preheat it at 360 degrees F, pour the eggs and salmon mix and cook for 20 minutes. Divide between plates and serve for breakfast.

Nutrition: calories 230, fat 12, fiber 3, carbs 5, protein 12

Peppers and Cream Cheese Casserole

Prep time: 15 minutes **Cooking time:** 5 minutes **Servings:** 2

Ingredients:

2 medium green peppers

1 chili pepper, chopped

4 oz chicken, shredded

1 tablespoon cream cheese

½ cup mozzarella, shredded

¼ teaspoon chili powder

Directions:

Remove the seeds from the bell peppers. After this, preheat the air fryer to 375F. Meanwhile, in the bowl mix up chili pepper, shredded chicken, cream cheese, and shredded Mozzarella. Add chili powder and stir the mixture until homogenous. After this, fill the bell peppers with chicken mixture and wrap in the foil. Put the peppers in the preheated air fryer and cook for 5 minutes.

Nutrition: calories 137, fat 4.9, fiber 1.2, carbs 3.5, protein 19.4

Mushrooms Spread

Preparation time: 5 minutes **Cooking time**: 20 minutes **Servings**: 4

Ingredients:

cup white mushrooms

¼ cup mozzarella, shredded

½ cup coconut cream

A pinch of salt and black pepper Cooking spray

Directions:

Put the mushrooms in your air fryer's basket, grease with cooking spray and cook at 370 degrees F for 20 minutes. Transfer to a blender, add the remaining ingredients, pulse well, divide into bowls and serve as a spread.

Nutrition: calories 202, fat 12, fiber 2, carbs 5, protein 7

Chicken Bites

Prep time: 15 minutes **Cooking time:** 8 minutes **Servings:** 4

Ingredients:

1 cup ground chicken, cooked

½ cup Cheddar cheese, shredded

1 egg, beaten

½ teaspoon salt

Cooking spray

Directions:

Put ground chicken and Cheddar cheese in the bowl. Add egg and salt and mix up the ingredients until you get a homogenous mixture. Preheat the air fryer to 390F. Spray the air fryer basket with the cooking spray from inside. Then make the small bites with the help of the scooper and place them in the air fryer basket. Cook the chicken and cheese bites for 4 minutes and then flip them on another side. Cook the bites for 4 minutes more.

Nutrition: calories 139, fat 8.4, fiber 0, carbs 0.3, protein 15

Tuna and Arugula Salad

Preparation time: 5 minutes **Cooking time**: 15 minutes **Servings**: 4

Ingredients:

½ pound smoked tuna, flaked 1 cup arugula

spring onions, chopped 1 tablespoon olive oil

A pinch of salt and black pepper

Directions:

In a bowl, all the ingredients except the oil and the arugula and whisk. Preheat the Air Fryer over 360 degrees F, add the oil and grease it. Pour the tuna mix, stir well, and cook for 15 minutes. In a salad bowl, combine the arugula with the tuna mix, toss and serve for breakfast.

Nutrition: calories 212, fat 8, fiber 3, carbs 5, protein 8

Cheddar and Ham Quiche

Prep time: 10 minutes **Cooking time:** 15 minutes **Servings:** 4

Ingredients:

4 oz ham, chopped

1 cup Cheddar cheese, shredded

1 tablespoon chives, chopped

½ zucchini, grated

¼ cup heavy cream

1 tablespoon almond flour

½ teaspoon salt

½ teaspoon ground black pepper

½ teaspoon dried oregano

5 eggs, beaten

1 teaspoon coconut oil, softened

Directions:

In the big bowl mix up ham, cheese, chives, zucchini, heavy cream, almond flour, salt, ground black pepper, oregano, and eggs. Stir the ingredients with the help of the fork until you get a homogenous mixture. After this, preheat the air fryer to 365F. Then gently grease the air fryer basket with coconut oil. Pour the ham mixture in the air fryer basket.

Cook the quiche for 15 minutes. Then check if the quiche mixture is crusty, cook for extra 5 minutes if needed.

Nutrition: calories 320, fat 24.8, fiber 1.6, carbs 4.7, protein 20.7

Coconut Eggs Mix

Preparation time: 5 minutes **Cooking time**: **8 minutes Servings**: 4

Ingredients:

1 tablespoon olive oil

and ½ cup coconut cream 8 eggs, whisked

½ cup mint, chopped

Salt and black pepper to the taste

Directions:

In a bowl, mix the cream with salt, pepper, eggs and mint, whisk, pour into the air fryer greased with the oil, spread, cook at 350 degrees F for 8 minutes, divide between plates and serve.

Nutrition: calories 212, fat 9, fiber 4, carbs 5, protein 11

Sausages Casserole

Prep time: 10 minutes **Cooking time:** 25 minutes **Servings:** 4

Ingredients:

3 spring onions, chopped

1 green bell pepper, sliced

¼ teaspoon salt

¼ teaspoon ground turmeric

¼ teaspoon ground paprika

10 oz Italian sausages

1 teaspoon olive oil

4 eggs

Directions:

Preheat the air fryer to 360F. Then pour olive oil in the air fryer basket. Add bell pepper and spring onions. Then sprinkle the vegetables with ground turmeric and salt.

Cook them for 5 minutes. When the time is finished, shake the air fryer basket gently. Chop the sausages roughly and add in the air fryer basket. Cook the ingredients for 10 minutes. Then crack the eggs over the sausages and cook the casserole for 10 minutes more.

Nutrition: calories 342, fat 27.9, fiber 1.7, carbs 6.3, protein 16.5

Almond Oatmeal

Preparation time: 5 minutes **Cooking time**: 15 minutes **Servings**: 4

Ingredients:

cups almond milk

cup coconut, shredded 2 teaspoons stevia

teaspoons vanilla extract

Directions:

In a pan that fits your air fryer, mix all the ingredients, stir well, introduce the pan in the machine and cook at 360 degrees F for 15 minutes. Divide into bowls and serve for breakfast.

Nutrition: calories 201, fat 13, fiber 2, carbs 4, protein 7

Chicken and Cream Lasagna

Prep time: 10 minutes **Cooking time:** 25 minutes **Servings:** 2

Ingredients:

1 egg, beaten

1 tablespoon heavy cream

1 teaspoon cream cheese

2 tablespoons almond flour

¼ teaspoon salt

¼ cup coconut cream

1 teaspoon dried basil

1 teaspoon keto tomato sauce

¼ cup Mozzarella, shredded

1 teaspoon butter, melted

½ cup ground chicken

Directions:

Make the lasagna batter: in the bowl mix up egg, heavy cream, cream cheese, and almond flour. Add coconut cream. Stir the liquid until smooth. Then preheat the air fryer to 355F. Brush the air fryer basket with butter.

Pour ½ part of lasagna batter in the air fryer basket and flatten it in one layer. Then in the separated bowl mix up tomato sauce, basil, salt, and ground chicken. Put the chicken mixture over the batter in the air fryer. Add beaten egg. Then top it with remaining lasagna batter and sprinkle with shredded Mozzarella. Cook the lasagna for 25 minutes.

Nutrition: calories 388, fat 31.8, fiber 3.8, carbs 8.7, protein 21

Turkey and Lime Gravy

Preparation time: 5 minutes **Cooking time**: 25 minutes **Servings**: 4

Ingredients:

1 big turkey breast, skinless, boneless, cubed and browned Juice of 1 lime

Zest of 1 lime, grated 1 cup chicken stock

3 tablespoons parsley, chopped 4 tablespoons butter, melted

2 tablespoons thyme, chopped A pinch of salt and black pepper

Directions:

Heat up a pan that fits the air fryer with the butter over medium heat, add all the ingredients except the turkey, whisk, bring to a simmer and cook for 5 minutes. Add the turkey cubes, put the pan in the air fryer and cook at 380 degrees F for 20 minutes. Divide the meat between plates, drizzle the gravy all over and serve.

Nutrition: calories 284, fat 13, fiber 3, carbs 5, protein 15

Thyme Chicken Meatballs

Prep time: 20 minutes **Cooking time:** 11 minutes
Servings: 6

Ingredients:

14 oz ground chicken

2 oz scallions, chopped

1 egg yolk

½ teaspoon dried thyme

½ teaspoon salt

1 tablespoon almond flour

1 teaspoon sesame oil

Directions:

Whisk the egg yolk and mix it up with ground chicken.
Add dried thyme, salt, and almond flour. Stir the mixture
until smooth and add scallions.

Mix up the mixture and make the medium-size meatballs. Use the scooper or make them with the help of the fingertips. Preheat the air fryer to 375F. Put the chicken meatballs in the air fryer and sprinkle with sesame oil.

Cook them for 7 minutes. Then flip the chicken meatballs on another side and cook for 4 minutes more. The time of cooking depends on the size of the meatballs.

Nutrition: calories 171, fat 8.8, fiber 0.8, carbs 1.8, protein 20.8

Almond Turkey and Shallots

Preparation time: 5 minutes **Cooking time**: 25 minutes **Servings**: 2

Ingredients:

1 big turkey breast, skinless, boneless and halved 1/3 cup almonds, chopped

Salt and black pepper to the taste 2 tablespoons olive oil

1 tablespoon sweet paprika 2 shallots, chopped

Directions:

In a pan that fits the air fryer, combine the turkey with all the other ingredients, toss, put the pan in the machine and cook at 370 degrees F for 25 minutes. Divide everything between plates and serve.

Nutrition: calories 274, fat 12, fiber 3, carbs 5, protein 14

Lemon Chicken Fillets

Prep time: 15 minutes **Cooking time:** 14 minutes
Servings: 2

Ingredients:

1 lemon pepper

¼ cup Cheddar cheese, shredded

8 oz chicken fillets

½ teaspoon dried cilantro

1 teaspoon coconut oil, melted

¼ teaspoon smoked paprika

Directions:

Cut the lemon pepper into halves and remove the seeds. Then cut the chicken fillet into 2 fillets. Make the horizontal cuts in every chicken fillet. Then sprinkle the chicken fillets with smoked paprika and dried cilantro. After this, fill them with lemon pepper halves and Cheddar cheese. Preheat the air fryer to 385F. Put the chicken fillets in the air fryer and sprinkle with melted coconut oil. Cook the chicken for 14 minutes.

Carefully transfer the chicken fillets in the serving plates.

Nutrition: calories 293, fat 15.4, fiber 0.1, carbs 0.4, protein 36.4

Basil Mascarpone Chicken Fillets

Prep time: 15 minutes **Cooking time:** 12 minutes **Servings:** 4

Ingredients:

1 tablespoon fresh basil, chopped

4 oz Mozzarella, sliced

12 oz chicken fillet

1 tablespoon nut oil

1 teaspoon chili flakes

1 teaspoon mascarpone

Directions:

Brush the air fryer pan with nut oil. Then cut the chicken fillet on 4 **Servings** and beat them gently with a kitchen hammer. After this, sprinkle the chicken fillets with chili flakes and put in the air fryer pan in one layer. Top the fillets with fresh basil and sprinkle with mascarpone. After this, top the chicken fillets with sliced Mozzarella.

Preheat the air fryer to 375F. Put the pan with Caprese chicken fillets in the air fryer and cook them for 12 minutes.

Nutrition: calories 274, fat 14.9, fiber 0, carbs 1.1, protein 32.8

Turkey with Cabbage

Preparation time: 5 minutes **Cooking time**: 25 minutes **Servings**: 4

Ingredients:

1 pound turkey meat, ground

A pinch of salt and black pepper 2 tablespoons butter, melted

1 ounce chicken stock

1 small red cabbage head, shredded 1 tablespoon sweet paprika, chopped 1 tablespoon parsley, chopped

Directions:

Heat up a pan that fits the air fryer with the butter, add the meat and brown for 5 minutes. Add all the other ingredients, toss, put the pan in the air fryer and cook at 380 degrees F for 20 minutes. Divide everything between plates and serve.

Nutrition: calories 284, fat 13, fiber 4, carbs 5, protein 14

Fried Chicken Halves

Prep time: 20 minutes **Cooking time:** 75 minutes **Servings:** 4

Ingredients:

16 oz whole chicken

1 tablespoon dried thyme

1 teaspoon ground cumin

1 teaspoon salt

1 tablespoon avocado oil

Directions:

Cut the chicken into halves and sprinkle it with dried thyme, cumin, and salt. Then brush the chicken halves with avocado oil. Preheat the air fryer to 365F. Put the chicken halves in the air fryer and cook them for 60 minutes. Then flip the chicken halves on another side and cook them for 15 minutes more.

Nutrition: calories 224, fat 9, fiber 0.5, carbs 0.9, protein 33

Cheddar Garlic Turkey

Preparation time: 5 minutes **Cooking time**: 20 minutes **Servings**: 4

Ingredients:

1 big turkey breast, skinless, boneless and cubed Salt and black pepper to the taste

¼ cup cheddar cheese, grated

¼ teaspoon garlic powder 1 tablespoon olive oil

Directions:

Rub the turkey cubes with the oil, season with salt, pepper and garlic powder and dredge in cheddar cheese. Put the turkey bits in your air fryer's basket and cook at 380 degrees F for 20 minutes. Divide between plates and serve with a side salad.

Nutrition: calories 240, fat 11, fiber 2, carbs 5, protein 12

Chicken Bites and Chili Sauce

Prep time: 15 minutes **Cooking time:** 10 minutes
Servings: 5

Ingredients:

15 oz chicken fillet

1 tablespoon peanut oil

1 teaspoon chili sauce

1 teaspoon lemon zest, grated

½ teaspoon onion powder

1 egg, beaten

½ teaspoon salt

Directions:

Cut the chicken fillet on 5 pieces and sprinkle with chili sauce, lemon zest, onion powder, and salt. Then dip every chicken piece in the beaten egg.

Preheat the air fryer to 400F. Sprinkle the air fryer basket with peanut oil. Put the chicken bites in the air fryer in one layer and cook them for 5 minutes from each side.

Nutrition: calories 199, fat 9.9, fiber 0, carbs 0.4, protein 25.7

Turkey and Coconut Broccoli

Preparation time: 5 minutes **Cooking time**: 25 minutes **Servings**: 4

Ingredients:

1 pound turkey meat, ground 2 garlic cloves, minced

teaspoon ginger, grated

teaspoons coconut aminos 3 tablespoons olive oil

2 broccoli heads, florets separated and then halved A pinch of salt and black pepper

1 teaspoon chili paste

Directions:

Heat up a pan that fits the air fryer with the oil over medium heat, add the meat and brown for 5 minutes. Add the rest of the ingredients, toss, put the pan in the fryer and cook at 380 degrees F for 20 minutes. Divide everything between plates and serve.

Nutrition: calories 274, fat 11, fiber 3, carbs 6, protein 12

Cranberries Pudding

Preparation time: 5 minutes **Cooking time**: 20 minutes **Servings**: 6

Ingredients:

1 cup cauliflower rice 2 cups almond milk

½ cup cranberries

1 teaspoon vanilla extract

Directions:

In a pan that fits your air fryer, mix all the ingredients, whisk a bit, put the pan in the fryer and cook at 360 degrees F for 20 minutes. Stir the pudding, divide into bowls and serve cold.

Nutrition: calories 211, fat 5, fiber 2, carbs 4, protein 7

Merengues

Prep time: 15 minutes **Cooking time:** 65 minutes **Servings:** 6

Ingredients:

2 egg whites

1 teaspoon lime zest, grated

1 teaspoon lime juice

4 tablespoons Erythritol

Directions:

Whisk the egg whites until soft peaks. Then add Erythritol and lime juice and whisk the egg whites until you get strong peaks. After this, add lime zest and carefully stir the egg white mixture. Preheat the air fryer to 275F. Line the air fryer basket with baking paper. With the help of the spoon make the small merengues and put them in the air fryer in one layer. Cook the dessert for 65 minutes.

Nutrition: calories 6, fat 0, fiber 0, carbs 0.2, protein 1.2

Lemon Coconut Bars

Preparation time: 10 minutes Cooking time: 20 minutes **Servings**: 12

Ingredients:

1 cup coconut cream

¼ cup cashew butter, soft

¾ cup swerve 1 egg, whisked

Juice of 1 lemon

1 teaspoon lemon peel, grated 1 teaspoon baking powder

Directions:

In a bowl, combine all the ingredients gradually and stir well. Spoon balls this on a baking sheet lined with parchment paper and flatten them. Put the sheet in the fryer and cook at 350 degrees F for 20 minutes. Cut into bars and serve cold.

Nutrition: calories 121, fat 5, fiber 1, carbs 4, protein 2

Orange Cinnamon Cookies

Prep time: 15 minutes **Cooking time:** 24 minutes
Servings: 10

Ingredients:

3 tablespoons cream cheese

3 tablespoons Erythritol

1 teaspoon vanilla extract

½ teaspoon ground cinnamon

1 egg, beaten

1 cup almond flour

½ teaspoon baking powder

1 teaspoon butter, softened

½ teaspoon orange zest, grated

Directions:

Put the cream cheese and Erythritol in the bowl. Add
vanilla extract, ground cinnamon, and almond flour. Stir

the mixture with the help of the spoon until homogenous. Then add egg, almond flour, baking powder, and butter. Add orange zest and stir the mass until homogenous. Then knead it with the help of the fingertips. Roll up the dough with the help of the rolling pin. Then make the cookies with the help of the cookies cutter.

Preheat the air fryer to 365F. Line the air fryer basket with baking paper. Put the cookies on the baking paper and cook them for 8 minutes. The time of cooking depends on the cooking size.

Nutrition: calories 38, fat 3.3, fiber 0.4, carbs 1, protein 1.4

Mini Almond Cakes

Preparation time: 10 minutes Cooking time: 20 minutes **Servings**: 4

Ingredients:

3 ounces dark chocolate, melted

¼ cup coconut oil, melted 2 tablespoons swerve

2 eggs, whisked

¼ teaspoon vanilla extract 1 tablespoon almond flour Cooking spray

Directions:

In bowl, combine all the ingredients except the cooking spray and whisk really well. Divide this into 4 ramekins greased with cooking spray, put them in the fryer and cook at 360 degrees F for 20 minutes. Serve warm.

Nutrition: calories 161, fat 12, fiber 1, carbs 4, protein 7

Chia Bites

Prep time: 15 minutes **Cooking time:** 8 minutes **Servings:** 2

Ingredients:

½ scoop of protein powder

1 egg, beaten

3 tablespoons almond flour

1 oz hazelnuts, grinded

1 tablespoon flax meal

1 teaspoon Splenda

1 teaspoon butter, softened

1 teaspoon chia seeds, dried

¼ teaspoon ground clove

Directions:

In the mixing bowl mix up protein powder, almond flour, grinded hazelnuts, flax meal, chia seeds, ground clove, and Splenda. Then add egg and butter and stir it with the help of the spoon until you get a homogenous mixture. Cut the mixture into pieces and make 2 bites of any shape with the help of the fingertips. Preheat the air fryer to 365F. Line the air fryer basket with baking paper and put the protein bites inside.

Cook them for 8 minutes.

Nutrition: calories 433, fat 35.5, fiber 7, carbs 15.6, protein 20.2

Espresso Cinnamon Cookies

Preparation time: 5 minutes **Cooking time**: 15 minutes **Servings**: 12

Ingredients:

8 tablespoons ghee, melted 1 cup almond flour

¼ cup brewed espresso

¼ cup swerve

½ tablespoon cinnamon powder 2 teaspoons baking powder

2 eggs, whisked

Directions:

In a bowl, mix all the ingredients and whisk well. Spread medium balls on a cookie sheet lined parchment paper, flatten them, put the cookie sheet in your air fryer and cook at 350 degrees F for 15 minutes. Serve the cookies cold.

Nutrition: calories 134, fat 12, fiber 2, carbs 4, protein 2

Turmeric Almond Pie

Prep time: 20 minutes **Cooking time:** 35 minutes
Servings: 4

Ingredients:

4 eggs, beaten

1 tablespoon poppy seeds

1 teaspoon ground turmeric

1 teaspoon vanilla extract

1 teaspoon baking powder

1 teaspoon lemon juice

1 cup almond flour

2 tablespoons heavy cream

¼ cup Erythritol

1 teaspoon avocado oil

Directions:

Put the eggs in the bowl. Add vanilla extract, baking powder, lemon juice, almond flour, heavy cream, and Erythritol. Then add avocado oil and poppy seeds. Add turmeric. With the help of the immersion blender, blend the pie batter until it is smooth. Line the air fryer cake mold with baking paper. Pour the pie batter in the cake mold. Flatten the pie surface with the help of the spatula if needed. Then preheat the air fryer to 365F. Put the cake mold in the air fryer and cook the pie for 35 minutes. When the pie is cooked, cool it completely and remove it from the cake mold. Cut the cooked pie into the Servings.

Nutrition: calories 149, fat 11.9, fiber 1.2, carbs 3.8, protein 7.7

Sponge Cake

Preparation time: 5 minutes **Cooking time**: 30 minutes **Servings**: 8

Ingredients:

1 cup ricotta, soft 1/3 swerve

3 eggs, whisked

1 cup almond flour

7 tablespoons ghee, melted 1 teaspoon baking powder Cooking spray

Directions:

In a bowl, combine all the ingredients except the cooking spray and stir them very well. Grease a cake pan that fits the air fryer with the cooking spray and pour the cake mix inside. Put the pan in the fryer and cook at 350 degrees F for 30 minutes. Cool the cake down, slice and serve.

Nutrition: calories 210, fat 12, fiber 3, carbs 6, protein 9

Olives and Eggs Mix

Preparation time: 5 minutes **Cooking time**: 20 minutes **Servings**: 4

Ingredients:

2 cups black olives, pitted and chopped 4 eggs, whisked

¼ teaspoon sweet paprika

1 tablespoon cilantro, chopped

½ cup cheddar, shredded

A pinch of salt and black pepper Cooking spray

Directions:

In a bowl, mix the eggs with the olives and all the ingredients except the cooking spray and stir well. Heat up your air fryer at 350 degrees F, grease it with cooking spray, pour the olives and eggs mixture, spread and cook for 20 minutes. Divide between plates and serve for breakfast.

Nutrition: calories 240, fat 14, fiber 3, carbs 5, protein 8

Cheddar Biscuits

Prep time: 15 minutes **Cooking time:** 8 minutes
Servings: 4

Ingredients:

½ cup almond flour

¼ cup Cheddar cheese, shredded

¾ teaspoon salt

1 egg, beaten

1 tablespoon mascarpone

1 tablespoon coconut oil, melted

¾ teaspoon baking powder

½ teaspoon apple cider vinegar

¼ teaspoon ground nutmeg

Directions:

In the big bowl mix up ground nutmeg, almond flour, salt, and baking powder. After this, add egg, apple cider vinegar, coconut oil, and mascarpone. Add cheese and knead the soft dough. Then with the help of the fingertips make the small balls (biscuits). Preheat the air fryer to 400F. Then line the air fryer basket with parchment. Place the cheese biscuits on the parchment and cook them for 8 minutes at 400F. Shake the biscuits during the cooking to avoid burning. The cooked cheese biscuits will have a golden brown color.

Nutrition: calories 102, fat 9.1, fiber 0.4, carbs 1.6, protein 4.3

Eggplant Spread

Preparation time: 5 minutes **Cooking time**: 20 minutes **Servings**: 4

Ingredients:

3 eggplants

Salt and black pepper to the taste 2 tablespoons chives, chopped

2 tablespoons olive oil

2 teaspoons sweet paprika

Directions:

Put the eggplants in your air fryer's basket and cook them for 20 minutes at 380 degrees F. Peel the eggplants, put them in a blender, add the rest of the ingredients, pulse well, divide into bowls and serve for breakfast.

Nutrition: calories 190, fat 7, fiber 3, carbs 5, protein 3

Fish Sticks

Prep time: 15 minutes **Cooking time:** 10 minutes **Servings:** 4

Ingredients:

8 oz cod fillet

1 egg, beaten

¼ cup coconut flour

¼ teaspoon ground coriander

¼ teaspoon ground paprika

¼ teaspoon ground cumin

¼ teaspoon Pink salt

1/3 cup coconut flakes

1 tablespoon mascarpone

1 teaspoon heavy cream

Cooking spray

Directions:

Chop the cod fillet roughly and put it in the blender. Add egg, coconut flour ground coriander, paprika, cumin, salt, and blend the mixture until smooth. After this, transfer it in the bowl. Line the chopping board with parchment. Place the fish mixture over the parchment and flatten it in the shape of the flat square. Then cut the fish square into sticks. In the separated bowl whisk together heavy cream and mascarpone. Sprinkle every fish stick with mascarpone mixture and after this, coat in the coconut flakes. Preheat the air fryer to 400F. Spray the air fryer basket with cooking spray and arrange the fish sticks inside. Cook the fish sticks for 10 minutes. Flip them on another side in halfway of cooking.

Nutrition: calories 101, fat 5, fiber 1, carbs 1.9, protein 12.4

Sprouts Hash

Preparation time: 5 minutes **Cooking time**: 20 minutes **Servings**: 4

Ingredients:

1 tablespoon olive oil

1 pound Brussels sprouts, shredded 4 eggs, whisked

½ cup coconut cream

Salt and black pepper to the taste 1 tablespoon chives, chopped

¼ cup cheddar cheese, shredded

Directions:

Preheat the Air Fryer at 360 degrees F and grease it with the oil. Spread the Brussels sprouts on the bottom of the fryer, then add the eggs mixed with the rest of the ingredients, toss a bit and cook for 20 minutes. Divide between plates and serve.

Nutrition: calories 242, fat 12, fiber 3, carbs 5, protein 9

Fried Bacon

Prep time: 10 minutes **Cooking time:** 12 minutes **Servings:** 4

Ingredients:

10 oz bacon

3 oz pork rinds

2 eggs, beaten

½ teaspoon salt

½ teaspoon ground black pepper

Cooking spray

Directions:

Cut the bacon into 4 cubes and sprinkle with salt and ground black pepper. After this dip the bacon cubes in the beaten eggs and coat in the pork rinds. Preheat the air fryer to 395F. Spray the air fryer basket with cooking spray and put the bacon cubes inside. Cook them for 6 minutes. Then flip the bacon on another side and cook for 6 minutes more or until it is light brown.

Nutrition: calories 537, fat 39.4, fiber 0.1, carbs 1.4, protein 42.7

Broccoli Casserole

Preparation time: 5 minutes **Cooking time**: 25 minutes **Servings**: 4

Ingredients:

1 broccoli head, florets separated and roughly chopped 2 ounces cheddar cheese, grated

4 eggs, whisked

cup almond milk

teaspoons cilantro, chopped Salt and black pepper to the taste

Directions:

In a bowl, mix the eggs with the milk, cilantro, salt and pepper and whisk. Put the broccoli in your air fryer, add the eggs mix over it, spread, sprinkle the cheese on top, cook at 350 degrees F for 25 minutes, divide between plates and serve for breakfast.

Nutrition: calories 214, fat 14, fiber 2, carbs 4, protein 9

Creamy Parmesan Eggs

Prep time: 10 minutes **Cooking time:** 8 minutes
Servings: 4

Ingredients:

4 eggs

1 tablespoon heavy cream

1 oz Parmesan, grated

1 teaspoon dried parsley

3 oz kielbasa, chopped

1 teaspoon coconut oil

Directions:

Toss the coconut oil in the air fryer basket and melt it at 385F. It will take about 2-3 minutes. Meanwhile, crack the eggs in the mixing bowl. Add heavy cream and dried parsley. Whisk the mixture. Put the chopped kielbasa in the melted coconut oil and cook it for 4 minutes at 385F. After this, add the whisked egg mixture, Parmesan, and stir with the help of the fork. Cook the eggs for 2 minutes. Then scramble them well and cook for 2 minutes more or until they get the desired texture.

Nutrition: calories 157, fat 12.2, fiber 0, carbs 1.5, protein 10.7

Buttery Eggs

Preparation time: 5 minutes **Cooking time**: 20 minutes **Servings**: 4

Ingredients:

2 tablespoons butter, melted 6 teaspoons basil pesto

cup mozzarella cheese, grated 6 eggs, whisked

tablespoons basil, chopped

A pinch of salt and black pepper

Directions:

In a bowl, mix all the ingredients except the butter and whisk them well. Preheat your Air Fryer at 360 degrees F, drizzle the butter on the bottom, spread the eggs mix, cook for 20 minutes and serve for breakfast.

Nutrition: calories 207, fat 14, fiber 3, carbs 4, protein 8

Sausage Bake

Prep time: 15 minutes **Cooking time:** 23 minutes **Servings:** 6

Ingredients:

2 jalapeno peppers, sliced

7 oz ground sausages

1 teaspoon dill seeds

3 oz Colby Jack Cheese, shredded

4 eggs, beaten

1 tablespoon cream cheese

½ teaspoon salt

1 teaspoon butter, softened

1 teaspoon olive oil

Directions:

Preheat the skillet well and pour the olive oil inside. Then add ground sausages, salt, and cook the mixture for 5-8 minutes over the medium heat Stir it from time to time. Meanwhile, preheat the air fryer to 400F. Grease the air fryer basket with softened butter and place the cooked ground sausages inside. Flatten the mixture and top with the sliced jalapeno peppers. Then add shredded cheese. In the mixing bowl mix up eggs and cream cheese. Pour the liquid over the cheese. Sprinkle the casserole with dill seeds. The cooking time of the casserole is 16 minutes at 400F. You can increase the cooking time if you prefer the crunchy crust.

Nutrition: calories 230, fat 18.9, fiber 0.3, carbs 1.3, protein 13.4

Spinach Samosa

Prep time: 25 minutes **Cooking time:** 20 minutes
Servings: 6

Ingredients:

1 teaspoon garlic, diced

¼ teaspoon ground ginger

1 teaspoon olive oil

1 teaspoon ground turmeric

½ teaspoon garam masala

½ teaspoon ground coriander

½ teaspoon chili flakes

1 cup spinach, chopped

3 spring onions, chopped

1 teaspoon keto tomato sauce

1 cup Mozzarella, shredded

½ cup almond flour

½ teaspoon baking powder

Cooking spray

Directions:

Preheat the olive oil in the skillet. Add garlic and ground ginger. Cook the ingredients for 2 minutes over the medium heat. Stir them well. Then add 1 teaspoon of ground turmeric, garam masala, ground coriander, and chili flakes. Add spinach and stir the mixture well. Add spring onions and tomato sauce. Stir the mixture well and cook it with the closed lid for 10 minutes over the low heat. The cooked spinach mixture should be very soft. Cool the spinach mixture. Meanwhile, make the samosa dough: microwave the cheese until it is melted. Then mix it up with almond flour and baking powder. Knead the soft dough and put it on the baking paper. Cover the dough with the second baking paper and roll-up. Then cut the flat dough on the triangles. Place the spinach mixture on every triangle and fold them in the shape of the samosa. Secure the edges of samosa well. Preheat the air fryer to 375F. Spray the air fryer basket with cooking spray. Put the samosa in the air fryer in one layer and cook for 5 minutes. Then flip samosa on another side and cook it for 5 minutes or until the meal is light brown.

Nutrition: calories 42, fat 2.8, fiber 0.7, carbs 2.6, protein 2.2

Parmesan Cherry Tomatoes

Preparation time: 5 minutes **Cooking time**: 15 minutes **Servings**: 4

Ingredients:

tablespoon ghee, melted

cups cherry tomatoes, halved 3 tablespoons scallions, chopped 1 teaspoon lemon zest, grated

2 tablespoons parsley, chopped

¼ cup parmesan, grated

Directions:

In a pan that fits the air fryer, combine all the ingredients except the parmesan, and toss. Sprinkle the parmesan on top, introduce the pan in the machine and cook at 360 degrees F for 10 minutes. Divide between plates and serve.

Nutrition: calories 141, fat 6, fiber 2, carbs 4, protein 7

Radicchio and Cauliflower Mix

Prep time: 10 minutes **Cooking time:** 15 minutes **Servings:** 4

Ingredients:

2 cups radicchio

2 eggs, beaten

2 oz Parmesan, grated

½ cup cauliflower, shredded

1 tablespoon butter, softened

½ teaspoon ground black pepper

¼ cup coconut cream

Directions:

Chop radicchio roughly and sprinkle it with ground black pepper. After this, grease the air fryer gratin mold with butter and put the radicchio inside. Top it with beaten egg, coconut cream, and Parmesan. Then add cauliflower. Mix up the mixture gently. Preheat the air fryer to 375F. Put the gratin in the air fryer basket and cover with the foil. Cook the gratin for 10 minutes. Then remove the foil from the gratin. Cook the meal for 5 minutes more.

Nutrition: calories 145, fat 11.8, fiber 0.9, carbs 3.2, protein 8.3

Butter Fennel

Preparation time: 5 minutes **Cooking time**: 12 minutes **Servings**: 4

Ingredients:

2 big fennel bulbs, sliced

2 tablespoons butter, melted

Salt and black pepper to the taste

½ cup coconut cream

Directions:

In a pan that fits the air fryer, combine all the ingredients, toss, introduce in the machine and cook at 370 degrees F for 12 minutes. Divide between plates and serve as a side dish.

Nutrition: calories 151, fat 3, fiber 2, carbs 4, protein 6

Thyme Zucchinis

Prep time: 10 minutes **Cooking time:** 12 minutes
Servings: 8

Ingredients:

12 oz zucchini, cubed

1/3 cup spring onions, chopped

1 teaspoon fresh thyme

2 eggs, beaten

3 tablespoons coconut milk

1 teaspoon olive oil

Directions:

In the air fryer pan, mix the zucchinis with spring onions and the other ingredients and cook for 12 minutes at 400F. Divide between plates and serve.

Nutrition: calories 54, fat 2.3, fiber 2, carbs 6.2, protein 2.6

Cream Cheese Zucchini

Preparation time: 5 minutes **Cooking time**: 15 minutes **Servings**: 4

Ingredients:

1 pound zucchinis, cut into wedges 1 cup cream cheese, soft

1 green onion, sliced

teaspoon garlic powder

tablespoons basil, chopped

A pinch of salt and black pepper 1 tablespoon butter, melted

Directions:

In a pan that fits your air fryer, mix the zucchinis with all the other ingredients, toss, introduce in the air fryer and cook at 370 degrees F for 15 minutes. Divide between plates and serve as a side dish.

Nutrition: calories 129, fat 6, fiber 2, carbs 5, protein 8

Balsamic Okra

Prep time: 10 minutes **Cooking time:** 6 minutes **Servings:** 2

Ingredients:

1 teaspoon balsamic vinegar

1 teaspoon avocado oil

8 oz okra, sliced

½ teaspoon salt

½ teaspoon white pepper

Directions:

Sprinkle the sliced okra with avocado oil, salt, and white pepper. Then preheat the air fryer to 360F. Put the okra in the air fryer basket and cook it for 3 minutes. Then shake the sliced vegetables well and cook for 3 minutes more. Transfer the cooked okra in the serving bowl and sprinkle with balsamic vinegar.

Nutrition: calories 50, fat 0.5, fiber 3.9, carbs 8.9, protein 2.3

Parsley Zucchini Rounds

Preparation time: 5 minutes **Cooking time**: 20 minutes **Servings**: 4

Ingredients:

4 zucchinis, sliced

1 egg, whisked

1 egg white, whisked

1 and ½ cups parmesan, grated

¼ cup parsley, chopped

½ teaspoon garlic powder Cooking spray

Directions:

In a bowl, mix the egg with egg whites, parmesan, parsley and garlic powder and whisk. Dredge each zucchini slice in this mix, place them all in your air fryer's basket, grease them with cooking spray and cook at 370 degrees F for 20 minutes. Divide between plates and serve as a side dish.

Nutrition: calories 183, fat 6, fiber 2, carbs 3, protein 8

Sage Artichoke

Prep time: 10 minutes **Cooking time:** 12 minutes **Servings:** 4

Ingredients:

4 artichokes

1 tablespoon sage

4 teaspoons avocado oil

1 teaspoon chives, chopped

½ teaspoon salt

Directions:

Cut the artichoke into halves and rub them with sage avocado oil, minced garlic, and salt. Preheat the air fryer to 375F. Place the artichoke halves in the air fryer basket and cook them for 12 minutes.

Nutrition: calories 84, fat 0.9, fiber 9, carbs 17.6, protein 5.5

www.ingramcontent.com/pod-product-compliance
Lightning Source LLC
Chambersburg PA
CBHW050748030426
42336CB00012B/1718